KILLING ME SOFTLY

By

Sharon J LeFevre

Sharon LeFevre is a B.A.(hons.) Drama graduate of Aberystwyth University of Wales. She is also a Self-Harm victim and now works in the field of drama and psychiatry, giving lectures and producing plays which she writes, directs and performs with psychiatrists and other mental health professionals. Her work as a mental health trainer, under the auspices and dedication of Ron Coleman, has enabled her to expand her own perceptions of what causes mental distress and how to enable professionals to have a better understanding towards their care of 'Users'. This is Sharon's first publication on Self-Harm based upon her experience and subsequent involvement with the work of A.C.T. (Action, Consultancy and Training.)

Sharon lives in Dolgellau in North Wales with her thirteen year old son. She has two daughters at University. She is currently working towards her Ph.D..based upon research using drama and psychiatry, in workshops and performances, to argue the pedagogical approach towards the teaching of psychiatry. This work is being supported by, A.C.T. (Action Consultancy and Training) Aberystwyth University College of Wales, dept.of Theatre, Film and Television and Ysbyty Gwynedd, The Hergest Unit, department of Psychological medicine, Bangor, Gwynedd.

CONTENTS

FOREWORD	R Coleman
INTRODUCTION	S LeFevre
PREFACE	The Provisional Order
CHAPTER One	Self-Harm what does it mean ?
Chapter Two	Computers Speak
Chapter Three	Language is Survival
Chapter Four	Doctors Orders
Chapter Five	Shrinking World, Shrinking Mind.
Chapter Six	Self-Abuse. Language and relationship with other.
Epilogue	Provisional Order Finale
Appendix	New Beginnings

FOREWORD

("Without Revolutionary Theory There Can Be No Revolutionary Practice")

Self harm and abuse are subjects which always cause emotions to run high, they are topics about which people find it difficult to be objective. Often when these subjects are tackled writers concentrate on the relationship between the abuser and the abused, or in self harm between the clinician and the client. Professionals often write papers which talk about the recovery of the self harmer in terms of the client stopping what is seen as self abuse. Practicing safe self harm is not seen as an option indeed most clinicians still believe that it is para suicide or attention seeking.

Rightly users who have written about self harm have concentrated on the subjective experience, relating in great detail the awful treatment meted out by a system that cannot grasp their reality. Users have demanded changes in the way they are treated in casualty and in psychiatry. Self Harm edited by Louise Pembroke was a milestone for users in that it took the debate onto new ground by defining users as the experts. This book together with the work of the Bristol self harm project began a process that is now unstoppable. The publication of Who's Hurting Who by Helen Spandler has added to this knowledge.

Killing Me Softly without doubt adds further knowledge to the debate. There is no moralism within its pages. Indeed it is the recognition of the contradictions that occur within abuse and self harm, and the controversy that this will cause which makes this book important. The author herself a self harmer has managed to remain objective about her own subjective experience throughout. Perhaps the most striking thing about this book is its no holds barred approach to the subject, which is at its best when the concept of recovery is discussed.

Killing Me Softly is not a comfortable read, and if you do not wish to be challenged then I would suggest that you do not bother opening these pages. The challenge posed by this book is a challenge to us all users, professionals and carers. If we accept this challenge then perhaps real changes in these areas can and will happen.

Introduction

The following pages may seem to the reader both shocking, disturbing and equally, they may even appear self-indulgent and irresponsible. As the reader you have the choice of which language you use to appropriate the text. As the writer and 'User' I can only give you my experience. I make no apologies for the explicit style with which I write and indeed ask for no approval. My aim is merely to endorse the experience as being 'real' and evidence of my 'truth'. The evaluation of this book however, can only be validated by your agreement to believe in my 'truth'. There is no hidden agenda and there is no scientific 'model' upon which I write, other than influence from my knowledge acquired from reading people. Therefore you will find this book sorely lacking in substantial references from eminent mental-health professionals. This is not by way of ignoring the dedicated and caring people who work constructively in research and practice within the field of mental- health. Indeed, my closest friends and allies come from the professional sector of mental- health. My most recent successful work is being carried out with the close partnership of Senior Consultant Psychiatrist Dr. Phil Thomas, himself well known for his forward thinking in psychiatry. His wonderful friendship and co-operation, performing alongside myself in my play 'On The Edge of a Dilemma', has been a source of inspiration and learning that I am ever indebted to. People like Ian Murray, senior nurse manager and active supporter of 'User' training is a man without whom, my life would be sorely empty. Mike Greenwood, senior nurse manager, a person who has shared some of my most traumatic encounters of self-harm, he has always shared my belief in its reasoning behaviour. Dirk Corstens, the Dutch psychiatrist who has become both firm friend and 'supporter' of my 'truth' is a special person in my life. Marius Romme, professor of the Dutch Limburg University of Psychological and Neurological medicine and Sondra Esher, scientific journalist, are people who have given inspiration and encouragement to myself and countless others. Professor Sashidhuran and Dr Christine Dean, Consultant Psychiatrist of Birmingham All Saints Hospital, have furiously enthused my work into their mainstream teaching for junior psychiatrists and their friendship is an enduringly important part of this work. Professor Alec Jenner, recently retired from psychiatry but still actively promoting research through conferences and the established 'Asylum' magazine. Dr. Terry Ogden my G.P. and trusted friend and allie who, always believing that I could achieve, initially set me on course for my university education whilst never turning me away in my times of extreme stress. Perhaps most important of all, my children, who have suffered immeasurable distress yet have stood by me and have never stopped loving me. Ron Coleman, a man whose bravery and dedication is an example to us all, is one man who does perhaps make it all, ever seem, ever possible. His care and teaching have not just given me a deeper understanding of the value of this work but it has also enabled me to believe in humanity again. These people and others, too numerous to mention, have in a sense, given me the route for the pathway along which I tentatively tread. The pathway is not yet finished and I hope that I will continue laying the stones upon which others may confidently follow.

Sharon J LeFevre 1996.

Preface

The Provisional Order

"I ask no questions and therefore, I tell no lies, yet as my 'truth' becomes 'me' it becomes one which the world denies."

The table is set, hand towel, tissues, larger towel for the floor, razor blades. I sit at *my* table, it is *my* table in *my* house. I have cleaned the house, I am very concerned that my house is clean; my chores are complete. I am up to date with the laundry, there is food in, the plants are watered. My son has clean, freshly ironed clothes. His room is tidy, my room is tidy. My work is up to date, I have completed all that I possibly can at this point in my life. Maybe I could have phoned someone, family perhaps, but I don't think so, not really, for that would mean talking, possibly telling lies and possibly being manipulated. I do not let external influences come in unless I am in a post-set state. I am not, I am in a pre-set state. I look at my watch, it is ten thirty p.m.. My son is in bed, possibly still awake *but*, he is fairly predictable, once in bed he nearly always goes to sleep.

I have cleaned my teeth, freshened up. I roll up my sleeve. I pick up the razor blade. It is a new blade. I rest my arm upon the table and I involuntarily flex my arm. I take the blade close to my plump flesh and it hovers there, waiting, as I decide to cut clean, un-scarred flesh. I then confidently guide the blade upon my upper arm, I position it, I do not hesitate and I carefully *slice it across, quickly, sharply!...* and a stream of red

blood appears, shimmers upon my skin. My heart beat increases, my breathing becomes deeper, louder, my teeth are clenched but there is only a loud melody in my head and like a demonic voice, it wails and urges, orders me to continue. I take the blade again, position the corner of it into the stream of blood and I press the blade down and *tear* it across the ready scratched skin. I pull it now and feel the flesh splitting open. Yes, I have broken through. I have opened the seal and now I must go deeper. The blade takes over now, my hand merely follows instructions. I cut again and *sure,...yes*, now the blood gets deeper, redder and it pours out and down my arm, falling suitably upon the towel on the floor. *No mess on the carpet please.* My eyes glaze over for a second, my ears thud and I feel momentarily faint. I lean down, steady my breathing. I hear the rain outside. I concentrate on the noise. My pulse is racing now and I must continue. *(I make a new cut, different place, just the same, must please everyone, can't be selfish, quick! quick! cut! Now go back to the first one.)* I am already feeling so much more energized, yet there is more to come, but I become more hesitant now for I know that I am going towards the *life* of me, the very...*life of me! I am getting nearer to a vein.* I take a new blade out of the wrapper, they are Gillette blades, always remind of men, certain men, *whom I know.* Another blade, it is sharper, fresher. I am going into deep territory now and possible pain but, try to do little sneaky cuts, just quick back and forwards into the open flesh. *I see the muscle splitting apart, see the tendons hovering there, and underneath I find the flow of the life force of my spirit, see inside my broken dreams and find myself and...Oh! A spurt ! A little fountain !*
I jump!
I mean, *I really jump !*

In shock!! An artery!! A little fountain of my blood!!

This is not about absent friends, not about *love* or *hate, money or poverty, success or failure!*. This is about 'time', the test of time and how much of it that we have.
The blood pours now but not so madly, freely as an artery, okay, just a bit deeper. *But suddenly!* No more!
Stop.
 Finish.
  Complete.

"My darling child you are so brave, so beautiful, so soft, so tasty".
Oh dear. I need!
Nurse ! I need some help. I'm cut open ... I need a....*oh*, I just, need !
My son, he's here in bed.

The doctor, he will call.

Twelve thirty p.m.. *tut, tut!* It's very late. Why are you on the kitchen floor bleeding ? Why,... *oh, why!*

Don't tell me off, please don't, don't, because you are my friend, aren't you ? You are my only contact in the cold pure hours of morning.

Stitches. Ought to be stitched ! Risk of infection, *tut, tut,* deep. What a shame!

Will you help ? Look after my son neighbor. I have to be sewn up.

God knows, ...*we don't want to be part of it !*

Just for now, I must stitch her up. Back soon.

Back now, sore, injection to anaesthetize. Good doc. Only, he gets mad, I see his look...*see his questions !*

Sore arm, sleep now, work tomorrow. *What shall I wear !*
Bandage is tight. Take it off. College tomorrow my girl.

Good!

Go to college. Son to school...*didn't see!* Kissed me good-bye.
Often says, "I love you !" not always, but often.
Good boy.
Love is all around him...*from me!*

        Of course... *he knows!*

Chapter One

'Self -Harm' What Does It Mean !

As A Metaphor ?

To find the 'self' there must be a representation upon which to locate the 'Self'. As Martin Buber said something like;

"To find the existence of 'me' (I) there must be the shaping/moulding of 'other' (You) "

How do we Shape ?

"I hear music my body begins to move to the rhythm of the music (Why?) because we are the music, (we) created the rhythm and therefore the rhythm is (us) it is intrinsically and culturally us! "

The consciousness of the identity is reliant upon the (universal) consciousness existing at all!

"To locate the consciousness of identity one must first be part of the already existing consciousness that is created by the identity of consciousness."

"I often feel conscious of having to click my (S)elf into the right mode of self, if you know what I mean. It's a bit like that game for children the one where you have to fit the right shapes into the right holes."

Fancy being so screwed up that you have to live your life working out why you are so screwed up !

"You live, you die,... and that's it."

No ! There has to be more! There has to be a source of energy that lives and breathes throughout the soul, that gives 'life' reason to live, to work, to love! There has to be.

"You live, you die... and that's it !"

There is a reason. There has to be a reason. You can't just exist. It's not just about existing! You have to feel that you are doing something, going somewhere, reaching out!

"Life is tough, nasty, ...and expensive."

"I have a blockage somewhere in my soul. It's as though I am trying to make contact and I just cannot get through. But if I let it get a hold of me, then I go crazy. It's like a dog chasing his own tail. Eventually you go mad because madness seems the better place to be. There is no pain in madness, there is nothing but oblivion, no guilt, no feeling."

Life is tough, nasty, and expensive !!

You must not let people use you for their own ends only to find yourself dumped by them. This is not love, friendship, loyalty. This is the exploitation of someone's vulnerability! People who behave this way are spoilt, selfish, greedy and insecure. They feed off vulnerable souls to make themselves feel good. Better to be alone than be treated this way.

Life is tough, nasty, and expensive !

No one is so powerful that one cannot break free! It is the duty of each individual to be responsible for their own actions and reactions.

Fear ! Fear and fear alone can drive someone into an unconscious state of security, *within the existence of that fear.* This *security* can be seen by those on the *outside* to be totally irrational, unsuitable and unhealthy. However, the person existing *within* this security, modifies the criteria of rationality and thereby creates their own stabilization of irrationality. In other words, their existence is bound up *within* the spectrum of fear; one that is ultimately dominated by the source (*instigator*) of that fear. In the long term this *irrationality* becomes a kind of protection from the fear which *ostensibly* keeps the person outside the 'reality' of that fear and, paradoxically, makes their life tolerable, sort of *fearless*. It is only when the person steps outside that *protection* that they become vulnerable to a rational awareness of their fear.

Why doesn't the person just go away from the fear ?

If we look at the natural instincts of the human psyche the most powerfully predominate one is that of the will to survive. Above all else it seems, the human being will, under extreme circumstances, fight for survival. To take an example, the maternal mother will instinctively put her 'young' before herself but if they are to survive from her protection then instinctively *she* must survive in order to carry out this protection. If we take this example and place it into the marriage scenario, where the mother's welfare is threatened by a violent partner, the mother's children will inevitably take priority over and above her own well-being. This ultimately means that she may suffer appalling conditions in order to maintain the status- quo of her family life. However, even if and when the conditions which she *(they)* has been living under are altered, the repercussions of this irrational yet rational *(to the mother)* state of fear may constantly resurrect itself into future relationships. In other words the fear can manifest in the person's psyche so that even when it has ended, the fear continues and may indeed induce the person to enter similar destructive relationships. The paradigm, sadly, becomes a way of survival.

(NB. This example can obviously be identified by either sex and to children in abusive relationships.)

Why ?

In tolerating abuse, once it has stopped happening, the abused person will have to go through, within the consciousness, a kind of spiritual healing. To heal one must at first be harmed and this is where self-abuse, paradoxically, becomes so ideal as a form of alliance for the abused person.

Alliance ?

Yes. To elaborate further, the psyche cannot respond to one single emotion. There must be, in a sense, a conflict of emotions going on for the individual to recognize that they are being abused in the first place. During the conflict signals are being registered. The abuse, once lived with and tolerated, became as it where a concept of 'truth' and, as was explained before, the 'truth' was reconstructed from irrational to rational so as to allow the toleration of the fear. Once the fear has been recognized however, through an external *interface* of rationality, the abuse becomes threatening to the 'truth' concept that was once recognized as *singularly* true. Now the 'truth' has been challenged by an alternative 'truth' and this also challenges the individuals conception of what is true. The dilemma then is one of being *damaged* by a misrepresentation of 'truth' and this misrepresentation creates its *own language!* The language is expressed through the self-abuse. The self-abuse becomes the internal arbitration that eventually emancipates the person from the misrepresentation of 'truth'. It is catastrophic in its resultant chaos, both physically and mentally even so, it is perhaps the only way for the abused person to survive.

Why ?

Well, the survival comes through the occupation of the abuse as a recognized reality. If the abused person were asked to dismiss the abuse then, in a sense, they are being asked to dismiss their own experience of reality. Reality is, in the philosophical sense, only relative to the person experiencing it. I *(me)* cannot experience your *(you)* reality. We share reality through the utterance of a shared concept *(understanding)* of reality.

"Who or what I am as far they are concerned,
is not necessarily, or thereby, me as far as I am concerned.
 I am presumably what they are describing, but
not their description. I am the territory, what they say I am is
their map of me.
 And what I call myself to myself is, presumably,
my map of me. What, o where, is the territory ?"

(R.D.Laing The Facts of Life.1976.p.27)

Chapter Two
Computers' Speak

"This is a table we both agree that it is a table."

If I say to you, " this is not a table it is an aeroplane," who is right and how do we know ?

Sorry ?

We know that I am wrong because our development our interaction is applied through a language, one that delivers a shared concept of reality. Without this shared concept of reality we would be unable to communicate in any sensible manner.

You mean, we both agree that it is a table ?

Yes. The table only exists within our reality because we both agree that it is a table. We do not question each others definition of the table because the language shared between us is the integral link to our communication. When we relate this analogy to sexual abuse it can help us to understand the complicity that takes place within the relationship of the abuser and the abused. In other words, if a child is being sexually abused and the child grows up with this language *(the abuse)* the child does not know that they are being abused. *(i.e.. this is a table we both agree that this is a table.)*

However, when the child becomes old enough to be aware of *another language,* through the child's development, the child has to reappropriate the first language. However, there is the now the problem of translation. *But, does the child translate or does the child become bilingual ?*

Translates !

Well, to translate a language the translation must accommodate a representation. For example, 'good' in French is *bien.* We only know this because while we are translating, we are *in transit* with our own language and we are rooted within cultural impasses that determine a meaning. When we translate a language we can only take it on good authority that what we are saying is what we are intending to say. To become bilingual however, means that one is learning *two* languages simultaneously. While I learn 'good' I also learn 'bien' therefore I am *rooted* into two cultural references, two frames of reality, through the adaptation of language. I do not need to translate from one to the other because I am rooted in both. I am both French and English. However, language subscribes to other complexities such as 'single language' translation that is only identifiable by its context.

Single language translation ?

Yes. I might say, " It is a glorious day today !"

What do I mean ? It might be raining and yet *I* think that it is glorious. If it is raining and I say this you might ask me what I mean by it because we have a mutual understanding that glorious means 'good' 'fine' 'sunny' weather. I then give a further explanation to make you understand what I am saying. It might be as simple as me meaning the way the light is catching the horizon through the sheeting rain. Or it might be that I am not even talking about the weather. To decide what I mean, initially, you would perhaps consider my mannerisms. For example, if I am looking up at the sky while I am breathily describing the *glorious day* then you would probably think that I do mean the environment in some way, or that I am mesmerized by thought. Or maybe I am being purposely vague or obtuse.

Language is a very complex phenomenon that for the most part is identified by our *shared* utterance being in a certain *context,* one to which we both - subconsciously, spiritually or pragmatically - aspire towards.

You mean, we agree ?

Yes. For example, if a right-wing politician and a left- wing politician say the same thing, they can be interpreting very different meanings based upon the ideology of their politics.

"People should not have to be reliant upon the 'state' for a decent standard of living."

The right -wing would seem to imply that people are *lazy* and the left-wing would seem to imply that people are being *exploited.*

Ah ! You mean, a table is not a table.!
Exactly. This frame of reference that we are in locates our spiritual existence (for there is no *factual* existence that we can *prove*) and denies 'other' (s) existence. Of course, political power is *based* upon such a philosophy of language. Control of this power is ordained and maintained through the

systematic subversion of language. If the political conflicts of the world were ever to be eliminated we would have to have one language and that 'one' would have to be similarly subverted to one contextual reference.

"Too much of anything is bad for you a little bit of everything is good," so say *all* of us.

An impossible achievement in any way other than oppression and that in a sense is not changing the language at all, it is just enforcement by political power.

But if we know that it works both ways then surely, we are making a choice of language?

Ah yes, but remember there is the 'power' circuit' to consider. The main frame of 'language' has inaugural power in that it can be manipulative and misrepresentative of what the original concept of its meaning is *(was)* to the receiver of the language. The *powerful* initiator of the language can subvert the language into alternative meanings, without actually changing its surface meaning. This powerful initiator of the language can use it to accommodate a private discourse between interlocutors *(people sharing the language)* and thereby distort any 'factual' definition of meaning.

You mean, 'love' is really 'hate' type thing ?
Well, yes, but it is not as simple as that you see, language is often defined by an *emotional* response. 'Love is really hate' tells us that love can be interpreted as hate but if we know it as love then, in theory, we should be able to see through this definition. But language abuse is much more sinister. Look

again at the politicians' example. They are actually saying the same thing, how we adopt/adapt the meaning is significant to our emotional preconceptions of the speaker and to our own reliance upon the speaker as a guide to our way of thinking. If we think of *language delivery* as if it is rather like a computer terminal we can try to work through the theory of power. There are several different sequences that one can use to go through to achieve what *ostensibly* appears to be the same destination, something on the screen., but what ends up on the screen however, may be very different from what was necessarily intended by its initial meaning. Information through language is ephemeral and elusive and is, in effect, part of the consciousness of the computer, it is part of *us* as we are that computer.

I will interpret this analogy to survival. The pathway to 'survival' is determined by the individual's *own route (the computer is fed information to get something up on the screen)* which is pre-determined by information. The destination is never actually reached of course *(what comes up on the screen is not fixed)* because, like the information on the screen , we can never actually know that when we get there it is the right place *(information)* to be. We can only be *there* within our own understanding of what *being there* means. However, we do not get anywhere alone, for as we understand, our existence is shaped/molded by our recognition and representation of 'other'.

Please explain this confusion !

Okay. If a computer 'expert' puts information into the computer, to gain information from the computer, then they are sharing a language with the computer, one that I may not have any conception of and of what, it means. The computer expert has a power over me, for my lack of understanding, but not over the computer for the expert relies upon the computer to share this understanding of language. If the computer expert fills up the computer with data that is not compatible then the computer will refuse to work but the computer only knows that it is incompatible by the fact that it has already been told what it will be compatible with. If the computer is stripped of its material however and is subsequently re-fed other information then it can be adapted to use different criteria upon which it will function.

Computers ? What has this to with Abuse ?

If a child is being sexually abused and does not know that it is sexual abuse the child is not *(in theory)* being sexually abused. Furthermore, when the child realizes that the abuse they are receiving is associated with their existence, through the actuality of the sharing; significance as an individual etc., then the child will have sub-consciously accepted this information as being intrinsically linked to their formulation of language. Ultimately the child will be dependent upon this information to form a certain *identi(kit)* of themselves. This identity then becomes dependent upon the abuse, in other words, the identity of the whole person is fixed within this terminal.

To diverge for a moment! The pleasure that we receive from 'love' for example, can equal the abuse which the child receives . To understand this further, looking at the language applied to the action can help. The English word for 'love' is *singularly* transcribed to several different definitions of love, i.e., parental love, passionate love, sibling love, filial love. Interestingly, the Greek words for love are separate in that they *differentiate* the type of love; the sexual, passionate love is *Eros,* the parental love is *Agape* and sibling or brotherly love is, *Phillipe.* If we think that *all* of our conscious understanding of love, in language, has to be pre-fixed by *action* before it is understood by the 'sharer' then the distortion of this love becomes more entangled within language than action.. If the child develops through the *action* of love, rather than through any contextual reference of what love means to the action, then there is a one way perception of what 'love' signifies to the receiver and of what it means in terms of, *connecting language with emotional responses received.* If there is physical pain connected to the lingual understanding of love through the love of a dependent *(i.e., a child and parent)* then the child only understands this physical pain being connected to love *(and not necessarily just to the person who gives it)* and to further this argument, the child is set up to respond to pain as an identity of love. If we look at how some parents and children greet each other in adulthood, in what can often be described as a robust and aggressive manner, we can more than likely determine that love is *(has been)* probably always displayed through aggression. Based upon the belief that the 'first love' of the human being is the pre-requisite of how *all* love is received and subsequently given out, then there becomes an elementary danger of 'misconception' as to the understanding of love through language.

Back to computers ?

Well, I am identifying the information in the computer as the 'abuse' to the child. The computer *(child)* understands the information from the computer expert *(abuser)* and a shared communication is obtained.

You mean sort of, X + Y = Z ?

Yes. The shared understanding of information *complies* with the desired result. The language used is exclusive to the interlocutors. This is the 'single language' translation by the abuser but to the young child it becomes the *only* language in use.

So it is not a choice of language then ?

No. At least not in the case of the young child. There is no comparison for the child to make, like the computer, the child is just fed the information. If the computer expert *(abuser)* presses the right buttons the computer *(child)* will respond accordingly.

Okay so what next ?

Next there is the learning growth development of the child into adult. The adult, by the natural course of development, inevitably becomes aware of *another language.*

No Computers ?

Well, if you like, it can be the 'virus in the computer time'. You see, the computer has been offered new information by another computer expert. This information is of equal relevance to the expert, as to what they would naturally feed in, but for some reason this computer spits it out, refuses to work with it, or maybe just keeps giving the wrong answers, because it is working on its 'Initial Response Theory'.

Initial Response Theory ?

Yes. 'The Initial Response Theory' is based upon the computer not being given the 'mutual' information that had been *previously* agreed upon. The 'virus' is the confusion if you like. It is not a refusal to acknowledge the information just a....

....Problem with Translation !

Exactly! The single language translation is not applicable to the computer *(abused)* because the computer *(abused)* does not have the knowledge of this translation process. If you like the new computer expert *(interlocutor)* is actually offering the computer *(abused)* an alternative view of the *package* that it has been using. Therefore you have the 'Initial Response Theory'. The previous expert had created their own translation of the computer language (the one that is shared by the computer package and the experts) but it only worked for them on the basis that they re-invented it.

What now then, I mean, people are not computers !

I am very glad that you said that because it is *here* at this point that we say good-bye to our computer analogy for a while. For it is *here* that we find the 'person' and the creation of the *intermediate language !*

Chapter Three

Language Is Survival ?

What is the Intermediary Language ?

The intermediary language is one that the abused person develops to cope with the confusion surrounding their single language and the new translation of this language. It is about, *survival !*

Why is it that the person cannot just accept the new language?

Well, the new language does not comply with the emotional responses that the person has been developed through. The new language is in conflict with the person's knowledge. This conflict creates a disturbance in the patterning of the person's development.

Patterning ?

Yes. Try to think of it as a dance.

A Dance ?

Yes. When you dance you move to a rhythm, a certain atmospheric rhythm. The rhythm is controlled by the music and the music is created by *you* in the sense that human beings are the only form of relative consciousness which creates the music in the first place. If the rhythm of the music is altered, your rhythm will be out of *sync* and you will be attempting to move against the rhythm rather than with it. The rhythm of your dance is thrown, aesthetically, speaking out of rhythm. Your rhythm becomes an abstraction from the *core* of the rhythm. If you do not understand the change of rhythm, due to a blockage in your atmosphere, then you are in effect in an intermediary state of rhythm.

Back to Language Please !

Okay. The intermediary language has to locate itself between 'two' other languages. To re-cap; the *first* language is *your truth, your reality,* the new language is someone else's truth, in fact, someone else's reality. The shock and complexity of recognizing that your *first knowledge* is in fact disagreed upon creates a massive mal-function within your terminal. For, like the *computer terminal* being dependent upon a shared language, you also are experiencing a break-down in communication. What is actually happening here is that someone is telling *you* that what *you* thought was 'truth' is in fact, not true! The effect of this dissociation from *your truth*, ontologically speaking , implies that you did not actually exist ! A profound and shattering experience for anyone to deal with. The result is that your expectations of existence have been nullified, obliterated and most importantly, denied of ever actually happening.

Just a minute, surely I would know that I existed by my own experience ?

Well, don't let us forget that you have just been informed that your 'concept of truth', *reality* was not true. Sorry, but back to the computer for a moment. The computer denies the new information because, quite simply, it cannot understand it. This is rather like a Word Perfect disk not being converted to Works.

Ah, right, got it. In theory then I am talking to someone who speaks Chinese when I don't!

Right ! Except that it is not just in theory it is actually in *your reality*. You do not understand this new language and therefore you are, to coin a phrase, "up a creek without a paddle". You are now, shall we say, in a in a state of flux, because, *a.* You cannot communicate with this new language because, as we have already established, you do not understand it, and, *b.* You have no one to communicate with in your own language, due to the fact that your *sharer* has presumably gone. Thereafter your existence, *reality,* becomes interminably threatened. To maintain your own sense of identity, which is of course essential to one's *sanity*, you cleverly create a diversion and through this diversion you create another language.

The Intermediary language ?

Right.

Self - Abuse ?

Unfortunately, yes. The self-abuse, *self-harm*, becomes a strategically dominant movement towards defining your own reality. The self-harm becomes the *proxy* of your *intrinsic* reality which you use to re-negotiate the existence of your 'truth', *your reality.*

So hurting myself becomes my way of understanding myself?

Yes. But it is also your way of maintaining your sanity and I am using the word *sanity* literally here and not with any flirtatious intent . For notice that I said *maintaining* your sanity and not reforming it, or denying that it exists. The self-harm, although seen by most professional carers of self-harm victims as an extremely negative and self-deprecating behavior, becomes the protection and surety of your welfare, your own care and control which will be maintained for as long as it takes *you* to realize that you can actually speak both languages and then choose which one you wish to speak.

So self-harm is a coping strategy or mechanism then ?

Ah! Well now that is a term often subscribed by the professionals that *in theory* seems a perfectly reasonable explanation. However, by using this term all it really achieves is time for the professional to work through a process of elimination; a very popular ethic in psychiatry, *generally*. But the danger here is that this use of *language* is both ambivalent and ambiguous, in that it neither creates an acceptance, other than a tokenistic one, nor does it reach beneath the surface meaning of the victim's intentions. In essence the irony of using 'coping strategy (*or mechanism*) probably ends up confusing the professional more than it does in assisting him in furthering any process of elimination. The dilemma is of course that professionals (*as do most professions*) need to have labels upon which to focus. This is understandable when you consider that the Freudian beginnings of psychiatry was calculated by evidential behavior based upon a 'label' of behavior and subsequently this popular method has remained intact. The 'behavior' needs to be explained, scientifically endorsed if you like, to allow it to become *psychiatrically* acceptable., hence the ambivalence. Furthermore, the *labeling* creates an immediate ambiguous interpretation, for by calling it a *behavior* (in the psychiatric sense) implies that it is mal-adaptive. But perhaps more enduringly worrying is that by using such a label as 'coping mechanism' rather pre-determines that the focusing of the professional will be concentrated upon this 'coping strategy' which limits the professional to a kind of 'spectatorship' rather than to an interaction with the victim. In other words the *focus* of the professional tends to lean far more upon the behavior than it does upon the person applying it. If we think of this as the professional actually interacting with the behavior -and this with a determined level of empowerment - it automatically restricts the liberation of the victim.

But surely, the professional is attempting to understand the behaviour to help the victim?

In essence yes, but let us witness what a tangled web results from this *understanding*.

<u>**Letters are sometimes the only way to find the words that you wish to say".**</u>

Dear Professional.

The other day when I came to see you in the surgery with two open wounds that I had inflicted upon myself, you said to me that you had better things to do than sew me up. I could not believe that you could be so hostile, so cruel, when you must have known how wretched I was feeling. If this wasn't enough you even told the nurse, *in front of me*, that I was a waste of your valuable time ! Oh, doctor, I do hope that you can sleep at night.

>Yours faithfully,

>Patient.

Dear Patient,
My training ,and subsequent practice of medicine, is about administering and *promoting* health care to the individual, who comes to me for damage incurred to their physical and mental well-being. If this *damage* is by self-infliction then it is beyond my capabilities to proceed with any external encouragement that would seem to cohere and condone such irrational behavior.

>Yours faithfully,

>Professional.

Dear Professional

Do you understand someone who beats his wife and then comes to you for treatment? Do you *treat* someone who eats too much food and becomes obese and then comes to you for treatment? Do you *condone* treatment for a person who drinks too much alcohol and then comes to you with a damaged liver? Do you tell the patient who has asthma and smokes that he is taking up your *valuable* time?

    Yours faithfully,

     Patient.

Dear Patient,

I must stress to you that anyone who purposely damages their own body has to be treated in a distancing manner. We, as doctors and medical professionals, cannot become an indulgence to your habit. As a learned behaviour it is beneficial to you that it is not recognized as an *acceptable* behavior. I do hope that you understand this and do not take any personal reference from my explanation.

    Yours faithfully,

     Professional.

Dear Professional,

When you are told by someone that you are a *waste of time* it very much initiates feelings of total loss and attachment to any self worth. Moreover, when it is a *doctor* who is telling you this, these feelings are heightened to the point of humiliation. Simply by the fact of being rejected from a recognized 'body' of professionals, upon whom you rely for their skills and expertise in the field of medicine, you are being denied your existence as part of the human race. My need from you was to stitched and that in itself is no less worthy of civility and kindness than any person coming to you for treatment. The fact that my wounds are self-inflicted should have no bearing upon your behaviour towards me other than in a way that might, understandably, provoke feelings of helplessness and distress. Treatment of the person is deserved of human kindness which, if not, *should be*, attributed to the reasons for a doctor taking up the medical profession in the first place!

Yours faithfully,

Patient.

Dear Patient,

I would suggest that you continue taking the prescription that I gave you and try to rationalize your behavior as a very negative approach to your getting well. When you establish responsibility for your actions we may see some progress.

     Yours faithfully,

     Professional.

Dear Professional.

I wanted to ask you a question the other day but you were so angry with me I felt unable to do so. I don't know why you pretended to anaesthetize my arm before you stitched it because the pain was absolutely incredible and I am *not stupid*. I have not been able to sleep for the last two nights because the experience is imprinted on my mind and keeps waking me up. It isn't like the pain of the needle going in and out of my raw flesh though, it is like the pain of rejection, the human rejection that I have never been able to forget from my life. In a way, you re-fueled that pain, the assurety that *this* pain of rejection and humiliation exists and, believe me, it is far more painful than cutting myself could ever be.

     Yours faithfully

     Patient.

Dear Patient,

I understand that your anger is unresolved, the anger from your past but, cutting or hurting your -self only creates more anger from people who are trying to help you, people such as my profession. Your responsibilities, as are all of ours, is to aware that you must learn to cope in a constructive and intelligent manner, one that may allow constructive help to be administered in a positive way.

    Yours faithfully,

    Professional.

Dear Professional.

When you ignore something it doesn't just go away it just moves to another corner. It still whimpers, it still cries, it still lives ! Don't you see ? The cuts are alive, they are a part of me, of my being! They don't just stop because you look the other way, they just bleed more heavily.

    Yours faithfully,

    Patient.

Dear Patient,

I am rather concerned about the amount of time that you spend in attempting to convince me that your self-harm is of benefit to me as a doctor. I can see only a temporary reliance upon this behavior as being beneficial to your acute stages of distress at needing attention.

> Yours faithfully,
>
> Professional.

Dear Professional

Who are you really, do you have children ? Are you married? Are you happy, do you get lonely, sad, do you like listening to music, *what type* ? Do you have happy or sad memories of your childhood. What newspaper do you read ?

> *Do you like cheese and pickle sandwiches ?*
>
> Yours faithfully,
>
> Patient.

Dear Patient,

I really find your questions quite unanswerable. It is not within my role as a doctor to discuss my personal life with my patients. I suggest that you should perhaps consider our relationship to be thwarted by the barriers of personal references. I further suggest that you consider our relationship as one of medical dependency, this way issues not related to your problems cannot interfere with your need for medical support. I really do not think that you should confuse yourself by seeing me as any one other than an administrator.

      Yours faithfully,

      Professional.

Dear Professional

I saw myself today in the mirror and when I really looked I saw you, I saw you looking at me. After all this time I am seeing not me anymore but you because your anger, your fear, your denial of me has at last been transmitted to me. You have done your job well professional, you have recreated me into your own image . Now I will go about my life with the same sense of well being as you have, one that denies humanity as being worthy of humanity. I will not be writing to you anymore professional because I am now a *professional.*

Yours faithfully,

ex-Patient.

"Hear my voice, child of the lost cause, stay within my reach and I will save you from the death of 'others' , those who deny your existence and only see you through their own, stay with me."

Yours,

The Voice.

These letters are very emotive but how do they deny the 'person' and only address the 'behaviour'?

Well, if we listen to the voice of the professional in these dialogues it is addressing the *behaviour*, as though it is a separate entity of the victim, when it is actually the 'script' that the victim uses to communicate between *present* self and self existing *within this present!* The reference to attention seeking, for example, is suitably flawed, because this ambivalence from the professional actually activates the *behaviour* as being separate from the victim and yet attached, in the sense that it becomes both barrier and arbitrator, according to the professional. However, this kind of 'spectatorship' from the professional is not unlike watching an actor performing on stage.

For example, if the actor is performing, lets say, *Hamlet* then the spectator believes that they are watching Hamlet but in actual fact, the spectator is watching the actor *playing* Hamlet. To play Hamlet the actor has to learn a script and has then allowed the *script* to determine that Hamlet actually exists (*on stage*). The actor still exists however for without the actor's consciousness you do not have Hamlet. (*The actor is always aware of himself- otherwise Hamlet would be learning his own script!*) The awareness of 'Hamlet' however, only transpires through the script and it is this 'tool' that enables the spectator to realize Hamlet. It is from this transference of information, from the actor to Hamlet and from Hamlet to the actor (*as Hamlet must be aware of the actor to make the actor exist*) that the existence of both appear on stage. If the professional relates the self-harm to the actor's 'script' *then* the professional will be relating to the victim communicating with the existence of their past and similarly their past will be *communicating* with their present, within the existence of the 'present'.

i.e., Actor relates to Hamlet. Hamlet relates to the Actor, through a script.

Victim(present) relates to victimised(past) Victimized(past) relates to victim(present), through self-harm(script).

If you deny the actor's (*victim's*) 'script' (*self-harm*) of having any agency towards these existence's and treat it merely as a superfluous kind of interval in the actor's (*victim's*) relativity, then the actor (*victim*) is without character (*identify*) to portray (live through). The actor cannot become Hamlet without communicating with Hamlet, *through a script!* In other words, if you deny the self-harm, the victim does not have a 'tool' with which to negotiate both 'past' and 'present' existence's of Self.

So you mean that the professional is watching a subjective experience. ?

Yes. It is actually an *intersubjective* experience which is linked by the self-abuse, the self-abuse is the actor's script. It is important to remember that with self-abuse there are an intrinsic set of rules being employed by the victim. These *rules* allow for discrepancies to be argued, for example, the victim can negotiate with the damaged areas of the past rather than just obliterate them (*which to do so would deny their existence*). Through this negotiation the victim can make allowances for these damaged areas but only by having control over them. This *control* is fundamental to any recovery. The recovery is fundamental to the victim finding status in the world. To re-unite with this world requires a learning process that enables the victim to identify with the *whole* self.

Ah! The actor has learned his script ?

In the sense that the actor knows his character and he can be Hamlet at *will*, yes. But to enhance on the above point, if the actor is not allowed to make his own decisions, as to how his Hamlet will walk, talk, frown laugh etc. then there will be no relation to his control over Hamlet, in fact it will not be his Hamlet at all. For a professional actor the performance would not only be unconvincing it would be superficial, for you cannot will the emotions they must come from some 'spur' within the consciousness. It is perhaps correct to add that it would be considered the Director's job to attempt to find that *spur* within the actor and of course *directing the actor* becomes the operative word here. Furthermore, it is the director's job to liberate the actor from the text. Coming off the book (term for actor learning the script) is the actuality of taking on the character. To take this argument further, it is impossible to enact a character without having personal autonomy over the manifestation of the character, the control comes from the conscious awareness of who the actor is playing. In other words, no two Hamlets' are the same. If we take this analogy and link the *professional* with the *director* then we can begin to see some relationship forming between the *victim* and the *professional* on a basis of mutual exchange. The problem of communication, for victim's of self-harm, merely invert when the professional tends to address the self-harm - lets say *'cutting'* - as though it is independent of the victim, i.e. **Razor blade verses Flesh.**

Professional- "I will not talk to you (*razor blade*) until you stop doing(*cutting*) that!"

Well, the bizarre side of this is that you do not get much conversation out of a razor blade (*the script lies upon the floor*) Talk to the victim *regardless* of the cutting and you might end up talking to someone who is a part of the victim's Self. The actor's director works through the script with the actor for many hours, weeks, months, before the script is ever finally put to one side (literally speaking). It is a process of *becoming* but *remaining* in harmony. The script cannot be worked upon without the actor and their character working *through* it.
(i.e. Hamlet to Actor/Actor to Hamlet . Victim to Victimized /Victimized to Victim).

So, these 'contracts' that are often suggested to patients, or are even insisted upon, do not work then ?

Well, this *contract* is a rather euphemistic way of saying "stop doing that and then we will talk" which is, in its utility, a rather condescending way of establishing *control* of the patient. Understandably the professional is probably scared and feels extremely vulnerable towards, the 'cutter'. But there is no clarification here of what is expected of either party. Is the professional suggesting that;

Not cutting is making the patient worthy of being spoken to ?
Not cutting is better for us to feel safe ?
Not cutting is my rule ?
Not cutting is allowing 'me' to address the issue of cutting in a sensible way ?
(The reader should note that these examples are not exclusive to 'cutting' it must always be noted that self-harm can be exercised in various different ways, as has been previously mentioned.)

Endless interpretations, none of which are particularly convincing. It is important to remember that the self-harmer is in charge of the Self not of *'other'*. The interminable *struggle* going on within the self-harmer is rather like a private party. (The) aggression from professionals can only reinforce the 'private party's' implicit belief of external hostility being derogatory to *their* well being; no uninvited guests here please! Professionals become exclusive with this *contract* (because they make it out and insist that you (*patient*) sign here) in the sense that the patient doesn't have any option, other to say no and then the professional will, perhaps as punishment, temporarily refuse further support until the next offer of the contract. Ultimately, this is not *helping* this is *bullying!* In fact this creates a divergence from the actual reason for the patient being in care and rather creates a whole new discourse between patient and professional. This discourse is not about care it is about challenging the concept of 'care by control'. The 'contract' becomes a tactic that is just another, albeit disguised, form of oppression for the patient. The idea of agreeing *not* to do something, on the basis of someone doing something for you, is denying a person of their rights by manipulative means. When you consider that the professional is supposed to be in the position of *care* and *compassion* towards the patient, a contractual agreement makes this care and compassion become quite an expensive commodity when it requires giving up your own power of thought.

But surely the contract offers a chance for the patient to attempt to give up the self-harm?

Self-harm is not *contractual* in the sense that it becomes something that you can give up on the basis of barter. Self-harm is an expression endogenous to the Self. It is more often than not referred to by *professionals* however, as an addiction or habit, neither of which are suitable definitions because they do not account for the victim's initial invitation to self-harm. If an addiction is understood to be some form of compulsive behaviour then such is life ! Of course, we know and understand that by addiction professionals are saying the person is doing 'this' to achieve 'that' result. What result ? Well, the answers to this question are manufactured to fit *the diagnosis of addiction.* If the self-harmer reports that they achieve a sense of relief from self-harming then this is immediately implied as being relative to addiction. On the basis of this kind of assumption you could say that emptying your bladder is addictive ! Furthermore, to comply with this kind of sterile diagnosis is nothing short of de-humanizing a person. The compliance of self-harmers towards this sense of reasoning usually happens through the victim's need for respite and support, sometimes everyone has to say (temporarily), 'if you can't beat 'em join em', just to gain some support. However, the self-harmer knows that they are just going along

with this *game* and that they will not stop self-harming just because someone suggests that they should !
They also know that this *attitude* of self-harm being an addiction or a habit is the epitome of ignorance.

<u>*In other words, hostility, aggression, alienation, from professionals merely compounds what has already been established , people do not care!*</u>

NB...The effects of such professional hostility inevitably lends its way into the mass market of media representation. The self-harmer becomes a subject of speculation by their family, friends, societies, communities. The 'risks' of becoming attached to the self-harmer are. to be seen as too great. The self-harmer is a non-person because self-harm becomes a label, a stigma and myths are thereby created. The self-harmer is deemed to be dangerous, weird, an embarrassment, unsuitable(sociable), irresponsible, masochistic. The damage ensued by the relationship of this language to the actual person can be irrevocable. The social rejection of the self-harmer merely reinforces the need for them to only rely upon the intermediary language (self-harm) to survive in a futile and hostile environment. Furthermore, once this language, used to define the self-harmer, becomes fixed within the professionals concept of the self-harmer, it automatically layers the victim's personality. But this personality is now being created by 'others' which inevitably becomes anchored into the minds of; trainees of mental health and general health medics, prospective employers, institutional bodies or organizations, and the general public. Once this discriminatory type of labeling is firmly stuck onto the self-harmer it causes the worst type of oppression imaginable. It is comparable to the most severe types of racial and economic oppression. The effect of this oppression, upon a victim's identity, can ultimately sever them from social relationships. Such severing from communal life often leads the victim into to sheer isolation, one which has a culminative affect upon their sense of self-esteem. It is often 'this' sheer isolation and alienation from people(!) and not the actual 'self-harm' that instigates suicidal tendencies, some of which are successful. It is simply not good enough (!) for professionals and 'others' to say afterwards (death of a victim) that the victim wanted to die. People do not 'want' to die, they are just left without choices !

But, going back to language, isn't the professional attempting to use the, 'intermediary language' ?

No ! The professional is attempting to *deny* the intermediary language by telling the victim to stop using it. This can only create delay in any progressive move forward towards the victim *choosing* a new language.

So there is a point of choosing then ?

In essence, yes, but it may take a *long time* for the emotional responses to collate enough evidence to determine that those choices do actually exist at all.

Why ? I mean if I know that they exist why can I not just take them ?

If only 'life' were that uncomplicated. Choices are made through the assimilation of experience and not just through facts. Supposing we take an example. If I say, have that car because it drives well and it is a good colour, do you have it ?

Possibly, if I take notice of what you say to me.

Yes, but you have taken notice of me and you do not understand me, *remember the Chinese !*

Yes, but if I learn Chinese then I can listen to you and take notice.

Listen yes, but take notice ? Not necessarily. Up to now you have taken notice of 'other' and you have been, shaped/moulded by 'other', *tricked, confused, shattered, humiliated, destroyed even.* Are you going to jump into another possible deception ?

So where do I go from here ?

                    To the next chapter.

Chapter Four

Doctor's Orders

I Must be Depressed ?

Unfortunately a lot of doctors will prescribe self- harmers (and this includes eating disorders, substance abuse etc.) with anti-depressants and neuroleptics when in fact very few people benefit from them and this is further clarified when comparisons are made to the number of people prescribed drugs. This is not to say that people do not benefit from them in the perhaps *acute* stages of their distress, as do many severely psychotic disorders from neuroleptics. However, this does not address or indeed excuse the irresponsible handling of drugs by our professional body of medicine. The 'medical model' of psychiatric treatment exercises complete *advocacy* of drug control over patients in psychiatric care. This 'drug treatment regime' is, thankfully, constantly being challenged by the more progressive *social* psychiatrists and 'user' groups and it is becoming recognized as a safer and more humane approach to avoid administering drugs. Ultimately, it is becoming popular to believe that to eliminate the individual's distress (i.e., the supposed illness) the professional must first learn to treat it, not as an illness but as a reactionary state of mind to the individual's reality. In other words, rather find alternative ways such as working with the traumas rather than against them and concentrate upon the *person* and not the symptoms. However, the administering of drugs is still considered by many professionals as being preventative medicine towards psychosis. Self-harmers' are often seen as psychotic because diagnosis is ambivalent when it comes to self-harm and anti-depressants and to some extent, neuroleptic drugs, become, in effect, just a sledge hammer to crack a walnut. This ambivalence towards self-harm is perhaps the most worrying aspect to consider when the self-harmer does become entrenched, within the system of mental -health care. For example;

Patient - *"Doctor I do not know why I am doing this !"*

Doctor - *"You are very depressed take one of these three times a day we will increase the dose as and when it is necessary."*

Patient - *"Okay. Thankyou doctor." (thinks) I'm depressed, that's what is wrong with me now I know.*

Are you suggesting then that depression does not exist ?

No. I am merely suggesting that using the term 'depression' is a convenient 'get out' clause for the professional to avoid searching for any fundamental cause for the victim's trauma. If the victim of self-harm has been told that their self-harm is caused by depression what *exactly* does this mean ? Depression is understood by a certain criteria that is established from what is believed to be the 'normal' functioning of a person. The 'depressive illness syndrome' merely becomes the medical (metaphorical) diagnosis of self-harm. It does not recognize the person beneath it (the self-harm) because it suggests that the person has been taken over by it (depression) In a way you could argue that this is what is happening but by prescribing anti-depressants as the 'cure' operative you are suggesting that the depression (self-harm) is separate from the person's consciousness which is like saying that the person has no control over her/his actions. Here we must make the distinction between someone who is *out of control* and someone who is *in control* of a distressing action, caused by something within themselves. If someone is out of control they will inevitably be taken into a safe environment and probably will need some form of drug support. If someone is in control of what appears to be a relatively unsafe action then calling it depression is not going to arrest it.

Depression can be a debilitating illness.

Yes, of course, if we *think* of it as an illness then yes, it is debilitating.

You mean it is not an illness ?

Well, if a person is extremely unhappy, afraid, lonely, confused about themselves, etc. etc. then they are not going to be *representative* of what we understand to be a 'normal' social - being are they, but this does not make them an *ill* person when using the definition of illness. It rather means that they are in a state of chaos.

Medication can help ?

Only in as much that it reduces one's *awareness* of this chaos and in that reduction of awareness, it obviously denies the person of the capacity to regain order from the chaos. Other than in the short term effect, of reducing the risk of the danger of the person losing control over their own sense of identity, medication is just a convenient and cost effective means of social-control.

Social control ?

The average doctor has an innumerable amount of patients and very little time to accommodate their needs. The only option for them in certain circumstances is to prescribe drugs that utilize the lack of therapeutic time that can be afforded to the patient. This can effectively reduce the amount of patient/doctor time that would be needed even though, the irony is that in the long-term, the patient often remains a 'patient' for a longer period. The doctor's administrative cost of their time to the health service can often deny them the accessibility to furthering the patients progress in any other than a prescriptive manner.

So 'getting well' is not cost effective ?

Not in the sense that the amount of time needed to accommodate some patients is more profoundly inhibited by administrative costs than by personal ones, no. However, all is not lost when the statutory institutes recognize that 'User' trainers are becoming more and more efficient at helping the statutory body of mental health to take some of the work load from them.

But Are The Professionals Aware of The Chaos not Illness Idea ?

Well, unfortunately not many admit to being aware, but yes, of course they are, but it would be more apt to say that they cannot be seen to be aware. You see, the general idea of illness is that it exists in its own right. It is not enough to say that depression, for example, is not depression but a compounded sense of irrationality towards one's own identity. Depression, like other mental health disorders, requires labeling. Each mental disorder is categorized and treated by reference to a model (criteria) of what the 'experts' propound as being suitably defined to fit the illness.

Do you mean, if the patient acts like this (x) s/he must have that (y)?

More or less, yes. There is, in effect, a deliberate criteria suited to adapt each individual's symptoms to the definition of illness. It is as crude as that but the prognosis of the individual's illness is left very much in the hands of the professionals' who are dealing with the patient. Of course, this can work for or against the patient, in as much as the prognosis is dependent upon the work ethic of the professional overseeing the case. However, even with slight variations of opinion the over- riding influence will always be that the patient is subjugated by this *illness* before they are recognized as a person in trauma. Moreover, the patient is denied access to any *argument* of this diagnosis simply because the 'experts' know best. Even worse is the fact that most patients, in their 'vulnerable state', actually feel *reassured* by a rigid diagnosis because it helps to maintain their 'identity in chaos' as an identity, which, paradoxically, helps to maintain its longevity.

The patient becomes paternalism by the doctor then ?

Yes, in a sense this is true because as a society we believe in our doctors and *their knowledge,* in contemporary medicine, is exclusive to them. Of course, doctors themselves are victims of their own success in that they do not question the *arbitrary* judgments that are made by *drug effective cures.*

Drug effective cures ?

Well, drugs *appear* to cure people, although the appearance is very often misleading in the sense that they reduce symptoms rather than cure them. The symptoms that the patient was *presenting* can be radically altered by drug induced states, but this merely suppression and not cure. What happens then of course is that statistics will provide *misleading* information. For example, a certain drug that reduces the patients dysfunctional behavior can seem to be an answer to the problem. If this information is multiplied, by statistical data, then the drug becomes answerable for the medical success. What happens then is that the drug will be highly recommended for use and will be saturating the market and will become the *doctor's* answer for treatment. The drug may have debilitating side effects and irreversible ones at that, but if it works upon the *surface illness* then this remains the compatible component to the diagnosis.

Are the doctor's acting in ignorance then ?

Not entirely, although using the word ignorance is probably misleading again, for doctor's are not miracle workers and just because they are doctors does not necessarily mean that they are good ones. They are, to a large degree, reliant upon the 'pluralistic' guidelines of medical knowledge to enable them to administer medicine. Don't forget, doctors' did not invent the minds of people they just invented their illness'. Their capacity to access and administer medicine *as individuals* is extremely limited and difficult to implement even if they want to. They are part of a 'body' the 'body' of medicine which inaugurates itself to the superior foundation of knowledge, of the human-being's state of health. The 'body' is represented by 'ethics' and 'principles' that are self-perpetuating and extremely difficult to challenge, unless you begin at the beginning again and change the way that they are taught. To do this efficiently of course, you have to break the chain reaction of this 'body' by impregnating it with challenging concepts and ideas that will flourish and not just be shoved to one side. It is slowly beginning to happen in mental health but more through public awareness and pressure groups than through the traditional 'medical body' actually wanting it to happen.

Why ?

Well, medical knowledge is a very precious and sacrosanct thing to have. It is rather like 'law' in that both of these *bodies* are representative of the 'human will' and its need for containment within society. The medical knowledge *supports* the knowledge of law and vice versa. The laws of medicine, especially in mental-health, become the fundamental pre-requisite for applying judicial law, in that madness is by design. Law enables medicine to function and medicine enables the law to be propounded. It is purely a matter of *decision making* from 'experts' as to who and what constitutes 'madness'. What is even more disturbing is that these 'experts' are very often people who have nothing what so ever to do with these respective institutions. The new 'Health Trusts' for example, are usually controlled by business people who have no knowledge of mental health what so ever! These business minded people are actually *in control* of making crucial decisions about where, how and on what the trust money is spent. The dependent area of health is therefore being organized, not by medical experts at all but by bureaucrats. This is rather like asking a garage mechanic to conduct the symphony orchestra, which, and let's be honest about this, would not produce a very tuneful composition.

These harsh realities are seriously impoverishing the chances of improvements in mental health care even with the shifts in perspectives. If we recognize that the mentally distressed are being deemed as mentally ill and are subsequently locked up like criminals and treated with abysmal attitudes of care then how do we define who is bad and who is mad ?

If I cut/abuse myself I am (not bad) mad ?

If I neglect my child I am mad (not bad) ?

If I murder someone I am not bad (mad) ?

How do you define what is right or wrong, mad or bad ? It is defined for us by some very powerful bodies. Once you become part of the body (i.e., the professional) you are part of this power and you are attached to the rules that govern this discipline of power. Power is not exclusive to the individual, it is only 'organized power' that is implemented by the individual, for no single entity of power can be exercised without the regenerative process of maintaining that power. Just think of your ability to empower yourself towards a raging bull. If you do not believe that you can physically overpower the bull you will turn away from him. The bull is more powerful than you are because it exercises more physical strength than you have. If a doctor wanted to refrain form doing a specified treatment and the patient relapsed or died, who is at fault ? The raging bull is the body of power that determines whether or not he will charge you. If he does then you can only run. If the 'medical body' deliver the franchise on how we live then we can only be subservient to it, or, we may just get crushed beneath it.

So, this is the 'distribution of power'?

Yes, in the sense that patients too have tremendous power but it is only operative in a collective sense, because the 'body' of medicine works on the probability concept that patients are less likely to enforce their power as individuals. You see, the poor old professionals' have a tough time too, which is why most of them prefer to have a quiet life and play by the majority rule. Not all doctors are pro-active in their work just the same as car mechanics, or landscape gardeners, some people do not question themselves, *ever.* To question oneself immediately limits your capacity to enforce power, because you become fragmented from the 'body' of the power that enables you to enforce in the first place. You are at once both impotent from the belief system of the mainframe of power and active in your capacity to *question* the mainframe of power.

It seems rather like a professional dilemma then ?

Yes, absolutely, in as much that professionals need their jobs and the empowerment of too many victims would actually create the redundancy of the professional

Where does this leave the patient ?

Well, it leaves the *victim,* for there are very few patients in mental health, in the world of 'victim status' which ultimately means that it is the victim who has to do most of the work. But to create victim empowerment we must at first recognize the world we live in as an ever changing evolving environment, one that will only remain in tact from recognized sources of moral behavior. Who defines this moral behavior however, is open to debate. You see, we are *all* victims of the environment and we *all* have to live within its capacity to accommodate ourselves.

Have we strayed from the subject somewhat ?

Not at all, in fact the next chapter exposes the wounds of the 'subject' if you like to put it that way.

Chapter Five

The shrinking world creates the shrinking mind ?

"There is a war going on, it is a silent war one that uses ammunition that is disguised as reality. This reality is utilized through a media representation of the Self. The Self must look think and feel in certain modified behaviors. It is designed by Experts who meet in secret destinations and spend many hours modeling the next, Self ."

" Sometimes I feel as though I am not really here at all that I am just a model of what someone expects me to be. "

Isn't this paranoia ?

Good question ! Paranoia is the creation of suspicion and people who are suspicious are generally considered to be a danger to themselves and to the society that protects them. But think what society is based upon and you will find that the fundamental pre-requisite for its survival is based upon a paradigm of paranoia. If we are not aware of what we are 'not' then we would not seek change and evolution would become merely a process of decay. It is through the *media representation* of reality that we do indeed become aware of what we are *not* and thereafter you have the creation of paranoia.

Doesn't this suggest that it is normal to be paranoid ?

If, by definition, paranoia means turning around and looking who is behind you then yes, for normality is, by definition, behaving in a manner that locates an awareness of how the majority behave.

Sounds rather abstract.

Well, let us look at the world that surrounds us, the one that is informed of its existence by the existence of its inhabitants. Globilization is the causation of the shrinking world through the eyes of technology. No longer does a person have to leave her/his domain to communicate with far reaching lands for we have an intercultural landscape upon which we all have a mat to stand upon. However, our *intra*cultural knowledge becomes at once exclusive and inclusive of 'other' because it no longer singularly dominates our pattern of thinking. We cannot escape this phenomenon so we have to defer to it but, historically, we are still linked to our own culture. The intercultural network however relies upon global economy and, thereafter, patronization of 'other'. We think that we are living reality when in actual fact *reality* is a creation of our own thoughts. The mind has to *shrink* into the global identity of this reality that persists as being the correct reality for our survival.

I feel paranoia coming on !

Well, the reality that we share is through this very realization of paranoia because survival instincts are about your environmental surroundings being safe for your own captivity. If you look at the great leaders of world affairs you will find that they are extremely suspicious people who are *cohabiting* within their 'intra' and 'inter' selves. If you scale this down to the single person's identity then you have an extremely vulnerable definition of what is (becomes) an identity (crisis).

Victim status ?

Right. The victim of humanity is about being someone who aspires to collude with what someone is *supposed* to be and not what you would *like* to be, or more importantly what you are (not).

Victims become the persecutors of victimhood ?

Absolutely. Take the example of the mother. She is reliant upon her own capacity to be a good maternal mother. She is told by *society* that she is a natural mother simply because she is the only human species who can reproduce. This is so concrete that there are even guide lines and books written as to how *experts* can ensure that the mothers' role is being fulfilled. When she has her child the mother should love the child and loving the child incorporates a whole work load of human responsibilities that are not even questionable as not being available from her because, of course, she is a *natural* mother. This burden to *love honor and obey* the demands of motherhood can have far reaching effects upon the mother's capacity to actually fulfill this role. The victim status of being a *good* mother then, subsequently, incorporates the victim status of what is expected of the child being a *good* child, which of course, is self-perpetuating. Disagreements between the two status' can involve some of the far reaching effects of mental health problems which often manifest in forms of ...

Self- abuse ?

Yes. For example, eating disorders. These are very much about a *relationship* between the food and the consumer of this food. The 'disorder' becomes the link that denies the consumer of food, which in turn denies the consumer of the right to consume. The relationship with the food becomes paradoxical in that it at once secures and prevents any real identity of any real relationship with the Self. If a mother has used food to give the fulfillment of love to the child, one that she may have been unable to give from herself, then the child has been reliant upon being *filled* as a substitute for love and possibly attention. The subsequent rejection of food, as in self-abuse, may be dependent upon the victim finding, not retribution to the mother, but the seeking of power towards regaining their identity. If we take the victim of the eating disorder as a person in their own right we find a rather confusing dilemma. Why does the person deny themselves of food and what does it achieve, other than serious distress and physical hardship. Well, let us suppose that the victim is using the food as a metaphor. This metaphor may be used in defining a previous relationship with another person, one who has obviously had a profound effect upon the victim. If this is so then we can begin to see that the food is synonymous with the 'other' person. The victim is not defining 'self' so much as 'self' is defining relationships.

You mean as a kind of strategy ?

Yes. The *eating* of food becomes a blockage towards locating any real feelings that the victim has had surpressed by relationships. The starvation allows the relationship to, in a metaphorical sense, die. The death is within the victim's consciousness and so allows the victim to take control of their emotional responses towards their own role in that relationship. In this way, although extremely distressing, the disorder becomes the positive relationship with personal empowerment. Bulimia is as similar to anorexia in that both deny and yet allow the 'self' to remonstrate with the 'self' about the emotional damage that has been incurred through the life of the victim.

Is this similar to the self-harm, cutting for example ?

The language phenomenon of 'cutting' is very similar to the food denial, or indulgence and then denial (vomiting). It is not at all unusual for self -abuse to include both or several of these disorders going on simultaneously, although victims tend to, in the chronic stage, address one act of self-abuse and stick to it.

Why does food become synonymous with 'self' and 'other' ?

Well, think of it as a strategy to survive amid a chaotic experience of emotional turmoil. We all know that food is the essential need for the physical self to survive. However, this *denial* of food is the challenge, to allow the mental self to evolve, to free itself from the barriers of the physical self. The *allowance* of sufficient food just to maintain the life of the person is the arbitrator if you like. The victim is conducting a kind of court scenario and they become at once judge and jury (and victim.) The judge is the food, *(how little do I need to stay alive)* the jury is the victim's own conscience *(you will not eat the more than I say*) the 'victim' deserves this torture to enable them to get back at 'other'.

How does this relate to the world image of Self ?

If we look at the media representation of how a person should *look* then we have a 'model' one to which we are expected to aspire towards. The *ideal* of this model becomes the consumer and the consumed, in the sense that one depends upon the other for its reality. The image sent out through this 'model' is extremely powerful when it is recognized as potentially successful. For example, if the young woman, or man, is to be slim, successful and envied then it must at first be the desire of the individual that motivates them to become this 'model'. The desire is implicit because the need to be accepted, within a society that dictates a certain criteria that is the recipe for acceptance, is created by ourselves. This is why advertising works. However, although the desire is implicit it is also exploitable for nothing is *fixed,* as is not our consciousness. Exploiting images of ideals then, becomes a way of distortion and our original ideal -one that may well have been accessible, reasonable - becomes distorted. Eventually, with mass induction the distortion becomes integrated in our way of thinking and, ultimately, in our way of *seeing.*
It is rather like taking a photograph of something that *you* see through an image of the mind's eye instead of the camera lens but one that is not *real* in reality, as though you have taken a picture and then touched it up to look how you believe it should look, rather than how it actually looks.

They say that people with eating disorders see themselves as fat when they are indeed emaciated ?

Yes, this is like the reversal of what the camera does. The person who thinks that they look fat is actually using this mental touching up technique because they are convinced that they are seeing the image of their own repulsion of identity. If you think of the 'mind's' camera lens as being arbitrary and the *actual* camera lens as being factual you are seeing two different images of the same thing. The question is, which one is real.

The camera lens ?

No. The camera lens gives out an image but the *mind's* eye translates this image into what the mind believes is real.

So the victim is right ?

In so far as *they* believe yes. The victim is the judge of what the jury delivers. The victim really does see this fat person.

So what is real then ?

Good question and it brings us right back to the idea of what is the *'normality'* of real. If the victim sees their own reality through the image of their own experience, one that has been related to food then they are living within their exclusive state of reality, one that cannot be shared by 'other' because it denies existence of 'other'. This is the traumatic chaos that pervades through eating disorders and self-abuse generally. Professionals tend to feel totally helpless when dealing with these patients. This largely is because they only really locate *illness* as the state of the person and not the relocation of identity, which of course is what is going on here. The professional will attempt to use drugs, punishment and alienation to force the victim to be sensible. This is both futile and dangerous for it merely denies the present experience of the victim (self - abuse) and more importantly denies the victim's reality of experiences.

Back to language ?

Well, it is the only tool that human beings have with which to communicate with themselves and others. Self -abuse is the language within the self and experience of the self and (the language with) 'other'. The language within the 'self' is like an exclusive language between the 'splitting of the self' and the two parts have equal rights. One is the 'self' acknowledging the self . As was explained before, there is a kind of private party going on and no outsiders can come in. The relation to 'other' then becomes a three-way conversation.

Chapter Six

If the self-abuse is language used through the image of the victim's 'present' life doesn't this have an effect upon their relationship with 'other' ?

"I am here for the interview, for the position that you have been advertising. You have my references, qualifications. I have also brought along some examples of my work. I am really excited about the prospect of working for your company. When I spoke to your personnel officer she sounded very positive about my chances of getting this position. Sorry ? My what ? My recent what...oh, yes, mental health problems, yes but they do not affect my...Sorry ? My arms ? Well yes, I know that they don't look so good but I assure you they do not affect...sorry...you don't have the position anymore ? Oh, I see, well, Thankyou for your time. I er..I'll see myself out..thank you...yes, of course, I quite understand..."

"Yes, I'd love to come to dinner with you. Yes, it is hot in here. My arms ? Oh, yes, I know they are badly scarred, I...you what ? You have to what ? You have to go, oh, right then I'll see you Thursday then at...sorry ? You'll call me ? Okay, ...but wait...you haven't got my number...I...I didn't give you my num...."

"You are a good friend, please, tell me, if you didn't know me, I mean if you didn't know me and you saw my scars, or someone told you that I self-harm what would you think, I mean would you employ me, want to have a relationship with me ? You'd probably think that I was what is known as a

*'nutter' and that I might just get a razor blade out at any time
? Oh right. You'd be scared of me, and you would be put off
having any kind of relationship with me. You wouldn't employ
me, not because you didn't like me, or that I wasn't competent
to do the work but because there is always the risk that I would
have a bad day. Oh, yes, but come on, I do not take sick time
out, in fact, I am as more or as less likely to get sick as anyone
I...you aren't talking about that kind of sick time ? No of course
I understand that you are talking about someone being
unstable. Oh, yes, of course I understand. Yes, of course I
know that you really like me. You sometimes feel embarrassed
introducing me to your colleagues ? No I didn't actually realize
this. Yes, of course I understand that it's not you who feels
embarrassed but that you have to think of how other people
see it. People who do not know me wouldn't understand it ?
Right, yes of course I accept that. You would expect people not
to want to leave me in charge of their children ? But I have
children I...You are trying to explain to me how the rest of the
world see people like me. Right, okay , how do they see me
and people like me ? As people who have something wrong
with their minds and that makes us different because what we
do is so horrific and frightening and that to the average
'normal' person it is unthinkable ? There is always the fear
that we might hurt someone else with the razor blade ? There
is always the problem of what you cannot see, (i.e., the
person's mind) and when it shows up in a mal-adaptive
behavior like 'cutting' or self-harm generally, it becomes
more obvious that you are a loony and the average person will
instinctively steer clear of you ?*

*Well, Thank you, you are a friend I know and I thank you for
being one because, of late, they have become somewhat
difficult to find.*

FACT !

People who have mental- health problems are marginalised more by the media representation of mental - health than by their actual ability to cope with their problems. This media representation is symptomatic of the sterile and reduced view of our world at large. The idea that people are able to go through their lives without experiencing emotions is the denigration of the human spirit and its resultant effect is that we create monsters rather than people. If we consider the atrocious crimes that are committed by some people, such as murder, rape, sexual abuse, physical and mental torture to another human being, we see people who 'should' be locked up in prisons. If we consider the people who are effected by these criminals and their subsequent crimes we find people who are locked up in prisons, prisons without walls, prisons that society has created by calling these people mad. The prison is of the mind, the mind of the public and their need to create madness out of despair.

Discrimination ?

The life style of the self-harm victim is, for the most part, isolated, introverted and constantly shadowed by the impending doom and despair of the *objective reality* of how their behavior is witnessed by the public.

Objective reality ? So they do recognize that objective reality exists then.

Oh yes, very much so. Victims of self-abuse are rarely so removed from their own trauma that they cannot relate to it in objectivity. In fact, this is often contributed to their trauma.

What do you mean, contributed ?

Well, objective reality exists *somewhere* for all of us, our conscious awareness is coded by it. Even so, there are many different views on what is, objective reality. If we believe that we subjectively can influence objective reality, i.e. that human beings can be part of changing the world , then we become intrinsically connected to that world.
Therefore, to 'live' one must at first be taking part in the *capacity* to live. This capacity is at once controlling and controlled by the unity of the individual's *placement* in the world. If this placement is denied by the manufacturing of a distinct *subversion,* towards any recognition of this placement, then the individual is being denied their own 'truth'. The concept of one's truth is the vital linchpin, if you like, to one's conception of existence. The only way to maintain that conception, when it is being denied, is to contain it within its (the truth's) subjective recognition. This further establishes the

argument that the victim of 'society' is most likely to be one who denies the *overruling* society, the one that dominates our lifestyle.

You mean, politically speaking ?

Yes, of course, for one cannot be apart from the politics of society even if one wants to be. But if the politics dictates that our life-style is weathered towards an objective reality, one that is not *our* idea of what objective reality should be, then there is resistance.

Towards the society ?

Well, it is never quite as concrete as that because the *society* is, in *effect,* resistance itself, this is why it dominates. To be resistant to society is to be resistant to the Self because, like it or not, we are *all* perpetuating the society by remaining within it. The politics of the society are woven into 'it' by people who resist 'it'.

Sorry ?

Well, if you do not resist it then there is no comparison to make towards it. For example, if all people ate the same food all the time and did not know of any other then it would not be questionable for debate as to; whether it is good for you, bad for you, tasty enough for you, distasteful or nutritious.

But you are talking about personal choices here, why could we not make personal choices ?

Choice can only be made when resistance is met. If one does not resist or to be more precise, defy, then there is no opportunity. If there is no opportunity then things remain as they are.

Confused !

Okay. If the victim of society (and we are *all* victims remember) can not challenge the resistance that he feels it will, in effect, become static, or stagnant. Politics work on the objective reality of the society. If I disagree with the political regime that I have to live under then I resist it and by resisting it I allow it to motivate me for if I did not resist 'it' I would be living 'it' without questioning it.

What is wrong with that ?

Nothing, except that as was stated before, it is impossible for *all* people to agree with *all* things at *all* times. The scientific approach in attempting to achieve this would be to laboratise everyone to *set* conditions (which is verging on 'normality' of course but I am identifying this in cruder terms). The philosophical approach in attempting this is to allow people to *be-come* instead of *be-made*. The reality is, however, that we are all dominated by a resistance.
A dominant force of power and control over us is created by their reaction to and awareness of our resistance.

Politics of the mind ?

Absolutely. Back to the victim's politics of mind and we have a resistance of the victim's politics, one that intrinsically denies him to be a part of a power that is(has been) controlling him. The resistance is to communicate with Self, or, in the case of objective reality (political choice) to exist in the objective reality that you are forced to live in by believing in the 'other' objective reality (which is created by resistance).

So how does the resistance maintain 'other'?

The resistance of the lived objective reality is 'here and now' the compliance to it is fixed 'here' but the resistance to comply (*e.g., strikes, demonstrations etc.*) makes it paradoxical in that because it is 'here', you resist it (*therefore you are recognizing its existence*) and it is (not)'there' because to resist you must have recognition of 'other'. If you agree to it then you are resisting 'other'(there) which equally allows 'other' to become a threat, which you must resist. Therefore, resistance creates and displaces one objective reality from the other, the changes are only met by force of dominance.

So self-harm becomes a manifestation of resistance ?

Right ! To take that away (resistance/self-harm) you must at first find how to replace it and what to replace it with. For example, you could not expect a Socialist to become a Capitalist without at first replacing the resistance of Capitalism.

How ?

Well, in a way this is what is happening in our world today. The fall of dictatorship or rather the shift of perspectives that created the fall of dictatorship was effectively due to resistance. The parliamentary left begins to redefine what socialism actually means and the Socialist begins to redefine his objective reality. Not in such an deferential manner that becomes derogatory to his beliefs and ethics however, but in way that allows him to, in a sense, re-create those ethics within the perameters that are feasible to him. Do not forget that ultimate power only comes from a *collective agreement* of that power and this is largely dependent upon external influences.

Why does he give in ?

He does not give in so much as re-focus because the balance of power shifts in such a strategical way that the original concept of his *objective reality* is no longer feasible and when this becomes obvious (*if only by its absence*) the evolutionary change over begins. Change is not a definite thing it is not a case of saying, *"I'm not going to do that or think this way anymore"* It is far more subtle and, thankfully, disagreeable. If let's say, all the water dried up in the reservoirs except for one, then everyone would *naturally* go to it - *to survive!* But if every day a gallon of water evaporated in one of the reservoirs and maybe four gallons dried up daily in the other two, then the shift would be less obvious but it would still be determined by the water, which is creating the reason to shift. The objective reality is changing but by such small measures that it becomes less noticeable. The dependency upon our objective reality is intrinsically linked within our subjective reality and vice versa, the understanding of 'both' relies upon a kind of radar system which permits us to hold onto our respective realities. Any interference within this radar system (i.e., the loss of water) will cause us to consider alternatives that are not necessarily a case of, *right or wrong* but just, absolute, in the fact that they are present.

Self-Abuse ?

Well, if someone suggests to the victim that the victim should stop the abuse, simply by order or punitive means then the response is bound to be a negative one because this offers no *reason* for the victim to stop. Indeed it will more than likely have the opposite effect because it nothing short of theft, in the sense that this *order* or *punishment*, is taking *abstracting* a part of the victim's (subjective/objective) reality. The suggestion to stop doing something, or believing in something, is an act of disempowering. Furthermore, it is the embodiment of oppression which *represents* the very resistance that this person is employing within their realities. In other words, the professional becomes the opposition and not the allie that he purports himself to be. The effects of such *psychiatric* oppression can be profoundly dangerous in that it (psychiatry) becomes instigator and not negator of the victim's reactionary tactics for survival.

There is no easy answer then, it seems not just frustrating but, well, sad ?

After the victim taking such vital measures, or to use the phrase, *'having the courage of your convictions'* the last thing that the victim needs to hear, about the order of their life is that it is sad. It is not sad, there is no sympathy needed here, there is perhaps a need for compassion, a need for medical attention when necessary and, of course, patience and understanding. Most importantly however, there is the need for respect, friendship, humanitarian consideration, for it is not *sad* but profoundly liberating that the victim has started to redress the chaos of his life. Professionals' *must* assume that their role is as a *facilitator* of support and alliance with the victim and not one of arbiter. The professional must meet the victim within the victim's territory, before they can expect to gain access to the victim's reality. They must not assume or approximate the victim by virtue of a paradigmatic eye. In essence, the professional must liberate themselves before they can expect to liberate the practice of psychiatry and ultimately their patients.

The walls of psychiatry seem to be impenetrably resistant to the social realities of people and yet they, the psychiatrists, are the idolaters of the mind, doesn't this seem rather contradictory ?

Let us be aware of the lives that people live. Doctors' go through a pre-emptive training for psychiatry that does not include a philosophy of the human-being but a biology of one. The transcript here is that the human being is a *body* before it is a living phenomenon, *a consciousness* of which there is no biological structure, other than an improvised one. The psychiatrist, therefore, comes upon the mind with a paradigm of its (the mind's) functional activity that is totally divorced from the patient's relative life experiences. The paradigm also pre-cludes any intervention of the patient's personal identity one that has been shaped by these life experiences. Doctors' are not people first, when confronted with a medical situation, they are doctors first. Take the surgeon. He has the skills that are needed to fix the body into a *functional* manner. He does not operate with the idea that the patient has a fundamental need for the diseased kidney which he is removing, he operates with the knowledge that the kidney is diseased and it is his job to remove it. The psychiatrist operates on the mind in much the same way. The difference of course is that he cannot visibly *see* the mind in the same way as the surgeon can *recognize* the kidney. Therefore the psychiatrist operates through an operative pattern of how the mind (supposedly) should function. He thereafter goes through the process of paternalising his patients with the security of his exclusive right to 'see' the mind. The kidney is the mind and the surgeon is the psychiatrist. The right to remove diseased parts of the body comes through the objective agreement between doctor and patient. In the case of the psychiatrist however, a sectioned patient loses his rights to determine his own mind. The *diseased* mind is taken over by the psychiatrist and the psychiatrist (and other mental health professionals) decide for the patient -through the behaviour of the patient and his responses to treatment - when this *disease* has been removed. The psychiatrist does not determine the patient's reality through his own he determines it through a paradigmatic one. In itself this pre-determines the patient's destiny as being held through the eye of the beholden (professional) and not through the beholders (the patient). The patient becomes a symptom of an illness that is a commodity. The psychiatrist is the consumer of that commodity. The patient becomes an 'it' rather than a person and so the cycle begins.

The cycle, but isn't the idea of psychiatry supposed to be linear in that it should move people forwards ?

I fear that the epilogue must come before the end for it is to this question that there is no answer.

If you are going on a journey and you know where you are going and you have planned this journey carefully then there is a good chance that you will succeed in getting where you want to be. Think about the journey though, in your mind's eye and think (see) all the possible things that could go wrong. Once you begin to work through all of these permutations they become infinite, in that their possibilities are never still and of course, if you allow them to affect your decision of traveling, you would probably end up staying where you are. This exercise is using the mind towards its capacity of thought. It is using your intellect to calculate and decipher. It is responding with your emotions to the possible problems that you might have to encounter. It is costing the effectiveness of your physical self. It is allowing an endurance test of your social and economic dependencies. It is instinctively weighing up your enthusiasm for the unknown. It is registering your capabilities as a pioneer. It is computing your knowledge against your observation. It is sighting your objective and concluding your aims. It is freeing your perspectives to work against the unknown quantity of your desires. But most of all, more powerful than any other force it is allowing your 'will ' to survive. This journey is the journey of life. For some people, who allow all these thoughts to integrate into the pattern of their journey, the traveling gets too rough and they have to take time out, find alternative ways of survival. These people are the mentally distressed. These people are living their journey every inch of the way.

A cure ?

Restore to health ? Get rid of (disease) ? Dictionary connotations of the word cure. Yet, realistically, *objectively,* before we can *restore to health* we have to agree on what the *shared utterance* of this word *health* actually means to us. If we at first look at the life of the victim before we decide upon the death of the person then we can work upon the fundamental needs of the victim.

Death of the person?

Well, if we see the cure as removing an illness and we decide that this *illness* is actually a person's identity then what are we doing ? If I am in a state of extreme distress, *self-harming* and you say that I am *ill* and you decide to eradicate my *illness* by denying me the right of *my feelings, my spirit,* then what else are you doing but, *'killing me softly'.* The 'victim' if you like, *is* the distress, trauma, *self-harm* that pervades the person's life and prevents their life being bearable. This reactionary behaviour, the *victim status,* is purely a protective coating, a layering upon the person's personality which allows 'time out' giving the person room to manoeuvre, *in other words*, the ability to survive amid a state of chaos. *Any* mental distress, I would go so far as to say, is a form of self-harm because it is the 'self' protecting the 'self'. You see, the paradox is that self-harm is not self-harm at all but self *protection*. Protection from what is recognized by the 'self' as a dangerous and hostile environment. Schizophrenia, or schizoid behaviour, is recognized by professionals as dysfunctional but it is only dysfunctional in that it prevents people functioning in the way that the world functions, *functionally.* If the body protects itself, as of course it does, *biologically,* then why should the mind not protect itself, *psychologically.* The behaviour of a schizoid person can be frightening, disturbing and debilitating for someone in the care of this person to witness. The very reason that we *need, have buildings* to cater for these people is to enable those who *choose* to work in this area of medicine, a place in which to do it. This may sound rather obvious but the experiences that many victims have of this care and support system are often horrifying to the extreme. Not only this but many victims are refused this chosen care, especially self-harm victims. They are refused on the basis of their conduct being unacceptable for the environment. The absurdity of this situation means that victims are literally thrown on the streets without support unless they *stop self-harming*. This creates immeasurable distress for the victim. Not only are they alienated by their own environment but they are alienated by the *safe* environment.

Why ?

The reasons are entrenched within the belief that by ignoring the self-harm the victim will become responsible for themselves and will stop self-harming. The myth, that 'to be good deserves favour' is relevant here but it fails miserably, because, once again, it denies the person and only recognizes the *victim* as the dysfunction. The dysfunction becomes the superfluous ailment and the person beneath becomes trapped within the rejection of the help available *and* the denial of their existence. The self-harm becomes the *only* available help to the person, the victim remains fixed, stuck in the role. The care from professionals is denied, the support from 'others' is denied because the *professional opinion* seeps mercilessly into the external support of the community. Eventually the victim's resources will inevitably come out in force *(the self-harm becomes severely dangerous)* and trap them into returning again and again through this cyclical system of *abusive* care. The extreme distress will often cause a victim to become sectioned and then put back into this sterile system of care that denies the person and speaks only to the victim. The victim is treated with aversion therapies. These consist of stitching cuts without anesthetics. Talking to the victim with hostile and patronizing attitudes. Shouting at and scolding the victim with humiliating and taunting attitudes. Refusing to talk to the victim when they are self-harming. The victim eventually learns new skills however, skills that enable them, not to survive their own distress but to survive the distress of the system of care. These skills are adopted by the victim as they learn that the professionals will respond to *good behaviour.* If a victim is recognized as seeming to interact more, on a level of *normality* i.e., wearing makeup, a smile, eating well, looking after their appearance, taking medication, taking an interest in hobbies etc., then the victim will be seen as growing, developing. The professionals' will feel a sense of relief and success. The professional feels smug and happy about their work. After all, the professional has achieved, with such ' abysmal treatment, a well patient. It is interesting to note here that most professionals will quite happily tell patients that at least seventy percent of patients *return* into the system time and time again. What is even more interesting is that they rarely seem to know why this is happening ! Their gratification seems to come from sending people out with a smile. But the smile is hiding the agony that the victim has come to realize exists, not only in their mind, but in the *system of care !* The professional may at times feel bemused by how well this abusive care works and they may even wonder at times (hopefully) if it is really the right way. Yet they will go on in this manner, regardless of any prick of the conscience because the they are trained not to be people but to be professionals. The professional has been told this is how it is done. It would be incredibly unfair to suppose that all these professionals actually don't care because their reality of caring is not at issue here. Most of them do actually admit to feeling mean etc., but they continue regardless because *well,* how can you care when the resources to care are not at hand and, *how* can you change things when no one really seems to know how to and *well,* as long as the function of mental health care keeps functioning, then you can only do what you can do and *well* that's it really and *well,* they are only loonies anyway.

How can the care improve then ?

The care can only improve by the re-thinking of what is perceived as self-harmful and what is perceived as self-protection. The professional must be re-educated in the practice of mental distress and recognize that their own resources are indeed limited. The professional must, in a sense, remove the barriers of the white coat and allow their own realities of personal welfare to come to the fore. The self-harmer, indeed, all mental distress, needs to be recognized as, not curable by design but by the will of intention. The process may be long and slow but it must begin with a recognized reality and not a designed one. The person is not the clothes horse that can be dressed in a biological garb, who is then sent out into the world and then be expected to *wear it well.* The designer label of mental- health has become old fashioned and cannot rely upon its buyers accepting bad workmanship anymore. The patient of mental health care has a right to expect that *care* just as the professional has a right to expect to have the means to carry out this care. When the professional accepts that the victim of self-harm is in need, of what we as a nation profess to be a high standard of intelligence within our health sector, then the care may begin to filter through in the appropriate manner. When the professional looks into the *world* for the reasons of mental distress, instead of into a *text book* then they might begin to find a person beneath the victim. The victim is the protection from the world and this world has to be replaced or the victim becomes non-existent the ultimate tragedy for some of these victims is suicide.

If people want to die though, what can the professional, or anyone, do ?

People do not want to die, they just run out of choices. The human body will survive until its resources to do so are destroyed. ***It does not destroy itself!*** All evidence shows that the human body protects itself. The mind will also protect itself. When resources run *out* so the mind does the ultimate in self-protection, it commits suicide. The harsh reality of *accepting* suicide, in the sense of believing that some people just want to die, is actually saying that *death* is more real to us than *life!* In other words, if we relate to the death of someone who commits suicide, as something that they wanted to happen, then we are believing in the reality of the person's death as being more *real* than the reality of a person's life! The effects of this are that we are training professionals to believe in death as an option. This kind of thinking, apart from obviously being extremely negative and morbid, is allowing the mind to escape into an unreal concept of what *living* is all about. The professional trainee comes into the profession of mental health with the realism of death, which in effect, negates life. It is not unusual, for example, to hear a professional or carer of a mentally distressed patient, to say that they would be better off dead. To hear this spoken in the corridors of medical hierarchy immediately pre-requisites the life of this type of person as being non-existent and the death becomes at once a tangible existence. If the trainee is being brought up with this kind of philosophy *(language)* then the reality of 'life' is being *sectioned, contained within a specimen jar!* Yet, worse its longevity is being challenged as desirable (or not) by its very fight for survival. If the person, who has become a victim, has their life assessed as *worthless* by the very people who are supposed to be helping 'it' (life) recover from trauma then what chance has humanity got to intervene. The suicide of any victim is *not* an easy option, it is not to be considered acceptable as a 'choice', it is to be considered the failure of a society to allow someone to lose the will to live. It is *unforgivable* to allow suicide to be dressed up as a 'choice' that was wanted by the victim. To believe this is to believe in a living person's death.

If we could rewind the film of the suicide victim would we still say that they wanted to die ? I fear not, for, like all re-winds we inevitably find something that we missed before. It is far too cowardly to say, " this person wanted to die".

"The end of this book, or rather this chapter, is only the beginning of the next, for never will the blood in my veins be still while my heart continues to beat and my mind thinks."

Sharon J LeFevre. Killing Me Softly. 1996.

The Provisional Order.

The table is set, it is my table in my house. The house is clean. I have cleaned the house. I always clean the house as I like it to be cleaned. I have finished the laundry. My son's clothes are washed and ironed. He is out tonight, he goes out with his friends now at weekends. He is working at the weekends so the money he earns he likes to spend. Sometimes he buys me little things, presents. I have to go to work tomorrow but its okay, because my boss, he doesn't mind. He knows you see, he knows that sometimes it happens. He'll probably find a reason to give me a hug or something, because he likes me to know that its okay, that it's okay. Then he'll say "get on with your work," in that kind of way when people pretend to be mad at you, the way that says, ' you are important to me because of who you are, not what you do!' I take out the towel, small one for the table, large one for the floor. I take out the blades and I lay them on the table. I roll up my sleeve and study my arm, look for a place that is not scarred. I find the option of my stomach might be preferable because my arm has been over used lately. I pull up my shirt and look at the flesh and I hold it firmly as I quickly take hold of the blade. I close my eyes for a second and I imagine myself sitting on a cloud in the sky serene and content as I feel the air about me, touching me and I am smiling. I open my eyes again and I see the blade in my hand and I know that there is work to be done. I breathe in slowly exhale and then and I put the blade to my flesh and I slice it firmly across the soft pale skin of my stomach. It immediately cuts through, the skin splits in two and I wince slightly because it feels...oh, I don't know, It just feels so open, so open! I look

at the stream of blood dripping out of the three inch cut and I know, I just know that I have to go again. I reach into the cut and pull the skin flat and I slice the blade through the broken skin and it falls apart, like a mouth opening, wailing. (part of 'me' cringes. part of 'me' wails.) **The blood oozes out and I quickly grab the towel before it runs onto my clothes. I feel unsure about this stomach area so I go back to the arm, the other arm perhaps. The voice urges me on and already I feel so much more energized. The blade has already reached my arm and my heart rate increases and I feel momentarily faint. I lean my head downwards and I hear the rain crashing down and I concentrate upon the noise. I look at my arm and I take the blade into the firm thin skin and I cut! Oh dear !**
It's deep!
It's deeper than I intended!
 It's bleeding heavily and I grip it tightly as a kind fizzy sensation shoots up my arm. Oh! Oh! I hope I haven't done it again, severed a tendon ! Oh no! Not again, please not again! I feel a little rush of tears then, just behind my eyes and then another moment goes by and they are gone again just as quickly. I dare to look at the huge gaping cut but, its okay, I think its okay. I think I will stop now, for I am tired, very tired, just very, very, tired.

You Draw Me in
   To The Aesthetic of Your Life. (written for Sharon, from Harry, a friend .)

THE END OR IS IT?

Introduction

When I began to self-harm I began to enter a new world. My life began to enter a new phase. It crept up on me, I mean, I had not been educated in self-harm. I new nothing of its history or logic, nothing of its language or rationale. It just happened, one Saturday morning in early December. I smashed a mug on the wall beside my bed. I smashed it with the intention of cutting my hand open. I succeeded, as you might expect with such a violent intentional act. It was not very serious, the cut I mean, but the intention behind it was, the intention was deadly serious. I was called upon by the local GP He was not my usual doctor but no matter, he was suitably concerned about my distress and the effects upon my son and daughter who were both in the house at the time. The amazing thing was that although every-one else was extremely confused and rather irritated by my aggression, I actually felt as though I had made contact with something, some *one*. I didn't know who of course or what, but I *felt it,* I felt it just as sure as I knew that this was only the beginning, the start of the journey.

Several years earlier I had made vain attempts to hurt myself. I had attempted to cut my wrists with a pair of blunt scissors, to scare someone, to show them some *part of me* that could not speak, that could not reach anywhere. I had played around with idle threats, to myself, towards taking an over-dose. Thinking back, I had often toyed with the idea of hurting myself in various different ways. Taking risks has always been my fateful attempt. Willing something to happen by the hand of fate. Dangerous pursuits have always been the challenge of the fear of me, the very fear of me coming to the fore of my extreme conscious desire to reach out, to touch the most impenetrable part of me. Have I wanted to die ? I don't think so not *really,* not really. I don't really believe that anyone wants to die, not *really.* I think that for us to say that a person *wanted* to die is absurd because how can we really know this anyway ? Just because someone says *it* does not mean that they really wanted it to happen. Maybe they want a certain part of them to die, the part of them that is causing them pain, unhappiness, severe mental distress, maybe they *do* want that part of them to die but not the whole of them, not the very *life* of them. Suicide attempts are usually made as a last resort, a desperate plea for help, a final demand if you like, to tell others that there is no other door open anymore but the door of death. Self-harm is far more sophisticated, controlled and safe in comparison. Self-harm, once learned, once the skill is perfected, is never deliberate suicide, if it is fatal it almost always by accident. So why do people do it ? *Why? Why,* when we love to show our-selves to the world, show our off our body in colour and variety of clothes and style, why do we inflict such terrible open wounding upon ourselves? Is it due to the age that we are living in ? Is it that we as 'a people' cannot speak anymore ? Is it that our mouths become sealed by the fear of hearing our own truth ? Or is it that we deny our own truth, that we bury it so deeply that we must eventually *cut* it out or *vomit* it out, or *starve* it out, just to survive. Self-harm becomes the destruction of the part that cannot stay inside that cannot bleed, cry, laugh, think, play. People say; "It is selfish!" "It is *violent!* " "It is attention seeking!" "It is *sickness."* "It is lack of intelligence, *insight."*

People ask; "Is it catching?" "Is it painful ?" *"Is it a turn on?"* "Is it necessary dear ?" "Wouldn't you rather hit a cushion ?" Well, maybe all or some of these comments are appropriate but even if they are, does that make the person wrong ? No! It makes the person *real* in as much as they are relating to this part of themselves.

I don't advocate it as a suitable survival programme, I mean I would certainly not encourage anyone to take it up, lets say, but I would not discredit it either, because the moment I discredit it then I discredit my own experience of life. In fact, the salvation of my experiences has been to self-harm. This may sound rather bizarre to those of you who only witness self-harm through another party. For those of you who are involved in any way with a self-harmer I am quite sure that you would rather hear less *positive* comments about it, especially form someone such as myself who works with professionals and users. But you see, there is no cure, there is no magic wand that any professional or family/care support system or person can buy, find, think of, make, adopt. There is no measure of alienation, isolation, punishment, trick aversion therapy that will succeed in doing anymore than creating reactions to suit the strategy employed. No, I am very sorry to inform you but there really isn't ! It is as straightforward as this, it is not curable by *design because it is not a designed behaviour!* Self-harm is survival and not suicide. If we attempt to provide a 'model' upon which you can attempt to cure self-harm then we are really wasting our time because medical 'models' do not address the cause they only address the symptoms. This would be rather like giving painkillers for terminal cancer and believing that the cancer is painless. It still carries on being painful cancer, it's just not recognized pain and then you still die. The person who self-harms can be threatened, they can be challenged, they can be confronted in much the same way as a disease is disguised but you cannot remove the person, just as you cannot remove a terminal

cancer. The person who self-harms *is* addressing the cause, the self-harmer *is* seeking self-help, the person who self-harms *is* tending to their wounds, wounds of the mind that no medical model can cure. To believe in such a cure is to insult the intellect, to humiliate the person into a non-person, a machine, a mechanical operative being. You cannot change what is quintessentially a part of someone but you can make it impossible to function and so, self-harm steps in, takes over and allows this quintessential part of someone to survive.
The decision to self-harm is not without its complexities of course, it rather takes its place in your life without invitation. It just becomes a way of communicating that forgoes approval. To the outsider it seems horrific, disgusting, and inevitably exhausting. It is all these things for the self-harmer. Oh yes, It is not all easy street being the chosen one to self-harm. There is always the down side to deal with. There is the hostility, the aggression and the fear. There is the ugliness, embarrassment and the pain and of course, there are the *scars!* The scars say it all really, when you really think about it, I mean the scars speak for them selves. They are perhaps the most *sordid* reminder of the fact that you are a self-harmer, as far as other people feel . You cannot blame people of course for the scars allow them no avoidance. For the professionals it speaks of failure; they couldn't stop this person harming their own body, they are the professionals and they have failed. Well, for the sake of all professionals I would like to express that you cannot fail something which you have not begun and you have not begun to fail a patient who comes to you with self-harm. You *fail* when you do not recognize that someone comes to you with an open mind. You *fail* when you ignore the person's open wounds, you *fail* when you treat this person as though they have no sense or rights. You *fail* when you deny the

person of their own experiences. You further fail when you turn the other way in disgust. For the family, friend, employer or who ever, being involved with the self-harmer, it is tough. I cannot dress it up, pretend that it is easy for them, it isn't. In the case of such people the self-harmer can only ask for patience, understanding maybe even a little compassion but if it is too tough then so be it for it is not *curable*.

What do we do then ? I hear you all shouting, what the bloody hell do we do ? Well, you could read this book again and you can ask yourself a few questions, questions like these;
What do I mean by the 'truth' ? What do I mean by 'reality' ? What do I mean by the 'mind' and how do I understand it as a sensitively, tuned, untouchable, yet vibrant 'thing' ?

The mind can, I believe, heal, but it cannot be eliminated, not by drugs or force or fear. It can *hide* and it can manifest itself in many guises but it cannot be eliminated, until of course, it decides to eliminate itself. To offer to repair something is to assume that something is broken. The mind does not 'break' it just dissipates its own awareness of experiences enough, so that it can organize the chaos, reset the sights and feed the starvation that threatens its very existence. ***The mind belongs to the person, don't steal it from them and just as importantly, don't ever deny them the right to own one, or you might just succeed in failing.***

Sharon J LeFevre. 1996.